Runaway Sugar

All About Diabetes

Dr. Alvin and Virginia B. Silverstein

Runaway Sugar

All About Diabetes

Illustrated by Harriett Barton

J.B. Lippincott New York

For information address J.B. Lippincott Junior Books, 10 East 53rd Street, New York, N.Y. 10022. Published simultaneously in Canada by Fitzhenry & Whiteside Limited, Toronto.
Designed by Harriett Barton

Library of Congress Cataloging in Publication Data

Silverstein, Alvin. Runaway sugar.
Summary: Describes the causes of diabetes
and what happens to the body when it occurs.
Also discusses symptoms and different kinds of treatment.
1. Diabetes—Juvenile literature.
[1. Diabetes] I. Silverstein, Virginia B.
II. Barton, Harriett. III. Title.
RC660.S557 1981 616.4'62 80-8727
ISBN 0-397-31928-2 AACR2 ISBN 0-397-31929-0 (lib. bdg.)

Runaway Sugar

All About Diabetes

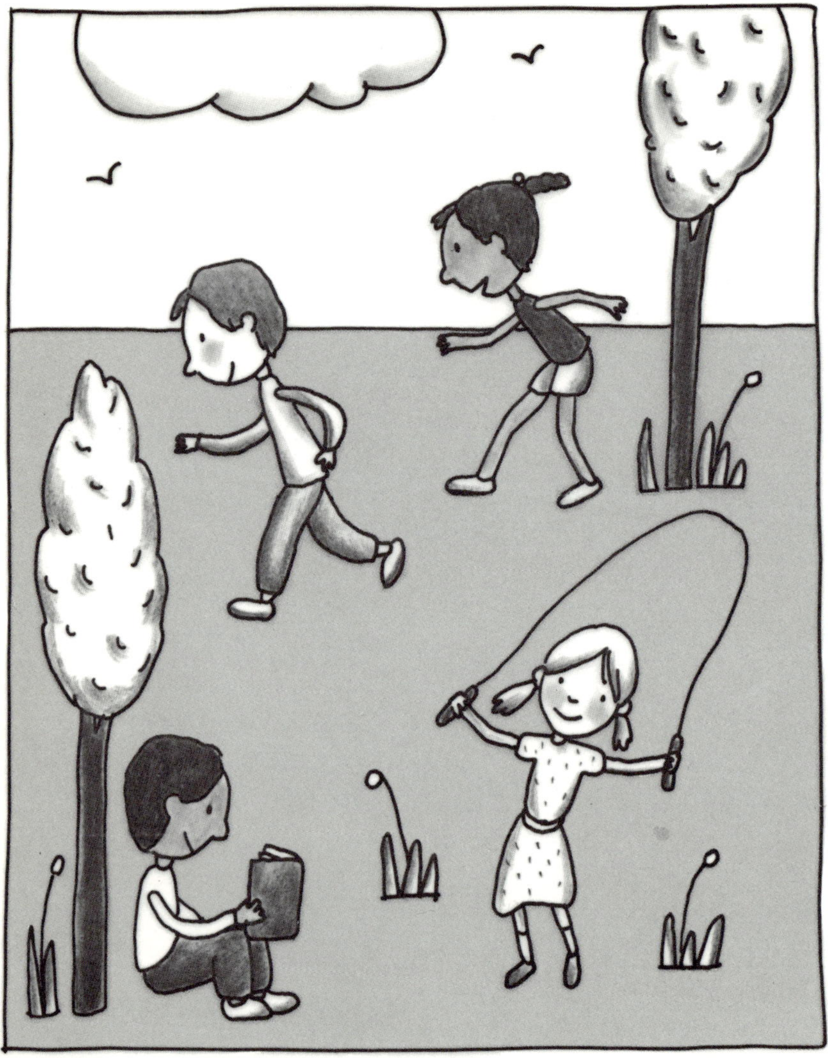

Do you like to play ball? Or jump rope? Or run races? Do you like to read books? Or draw pictures?

All these things can be fun. But they all take energy.

A car needs energy to make it go. It gets its energy from gasoline. The gasoline is burned in the car's engine.

People get their energy from foods. The foods we eat are "burned" too. But it is a different kind of burning. It is much slower and steadier. A fire gives out a lot of energy, all at once. But our bodies can get energy from foods a little at a time, as it is needed.

Sugars are one kind of energy food. How much sugar do you eat? There is sugar in jam and jelly. There is sugar in honey and syrup. There is sugar in fruit. Candy and soda drinks are full of sugar.

The body can also use starches for energy. First it must change the starches into sugars. It is a little slower getting energy that way. But starches are good energy foods. There is a lot of starch in bread. There is starch in cereal, too. Spaghetti and potatoes also have plenty of starch.

We can also get energy from fats. Fats are found in butter, margarine, oils, and the fatty parts of meat.

Meat contains a lot of another kind of food, called protein. The body can get energy from protein. More often protein is used for building muscles and other body parts. You need plenty of protein when you are growing. But even when you are grown up, you will still need protein to keep you healthy and strong.

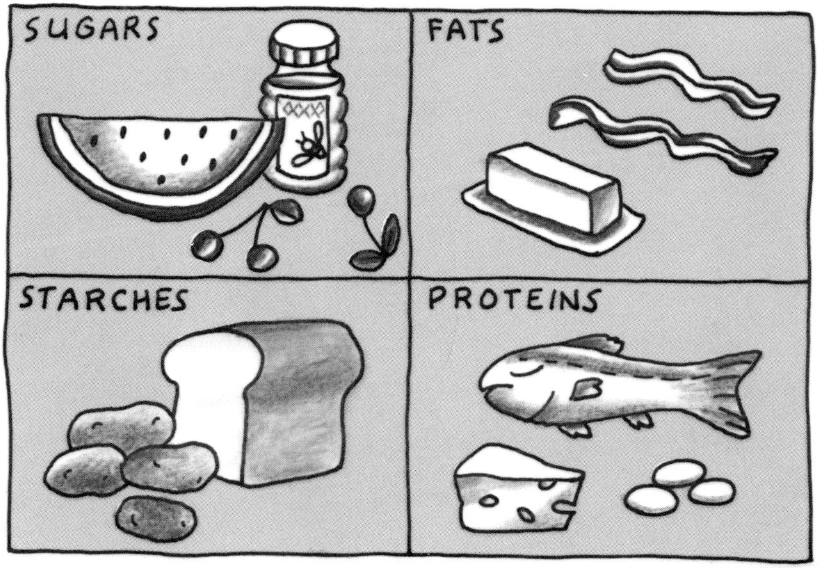

Sometimes the body uses protein as an energy food. But usually we get our energy mainly from sugars and starches.

Some special chemicals are needed for the body to get energy from sugar. These chemicals are called hormones. They are made in organs called glands. Hormones pass through the thin walls of tiny blood vessels into the blood. The blood carries hormones all through the body.

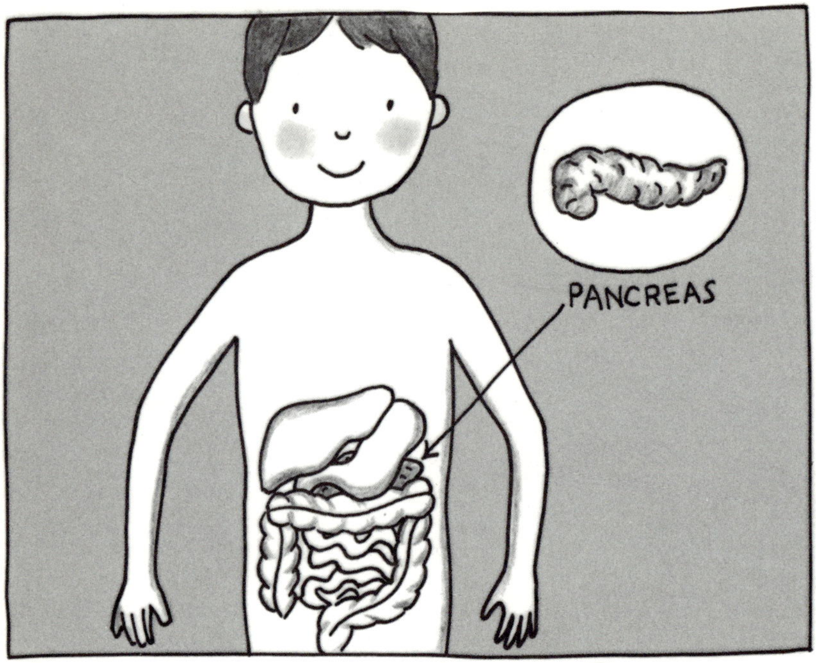

A gland called the pancreas makes hormones that help in getting and using energy. The pancreas lies just under the stomach. It is shaped something like a fish. Two of its hormones are called insulin and glucagon. These hormones are produced all the time, but their amounts depend on how much sugar is in the blood.

When there is too much sugar in the blood, the pancreas makes more insulin. Insulin makes the blood sugar level go down.

If there is not enough sugar in the blood, the pancreas makes more glucagon. Glucagon makes the blood sugar level go up.

Insulin and glucagon work together like members of a team. They make sure that the amount of sugar in the blood is always just right.

How do insulin and glucagon work?

After you eat, the foods are digested in your stomach and intestines. (That is where the starches are changed into sugars.) Sugars and other food materials pass into your blood. Insulin makes sugar go out of the blood into the cells of the body. Some cells change the sugar into a kind of "animal starch," which is a handy form for storing this energy food. (The liver is the main sugar storer in the body.) Other cells change sugar into fats. The cells hold onto the animal starch or fat until the body

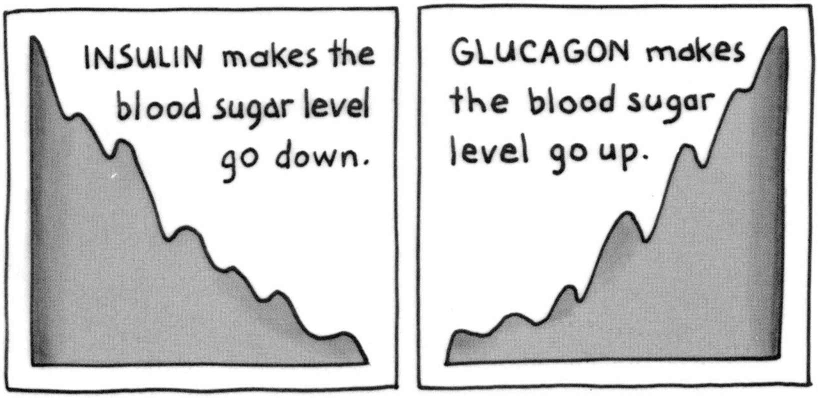

needs some extra energy.

Glucagon makes animal starch in the cells turn back into sugar. The sugar goes into the blood. It is carried to the cells that need energy.

If there were not enough sugar in your blood, you would feel sick. Your cells could not get enough energy. You couldn't think straight. You would feel tired. You might faint.

Too much sugar in your blood could also make you sick. If the sugar stayed in the blood, then the cells could not burn it for energy. They would have to burn something else. They might use the protein from your muscles. But then you would get weak. They might use fats for energy. When fats are burned, they give a lot of energy. But they also form chemicals called ketone bodies. Too many ketone bodies can poison cells. They can harm the body.

Some people have too much sugar in their blood. They suffer from a disease called diabetes.

Five million people in the United States are now being treated for diabetes. Doctors suspect that another five million have the disease but don't know it. Each new baby that is born has about one chance in ten of getting diabetes someday.

Most people who have diabetes are middle-aged or old. But children—even babies—can also get this disease. The kind of diabetes that children get is called juvenile diabetes, or insulin dependent diabetes. It is often much worse than the kind that strikes adults. Juvenile diabetes may start very suddenly, and it can be a very serious illness.

What causes diabetes? Doctors and scientists don't have all the answers yet. But they have learned a lot about this disease, and they are learning more all the time.

Scientists now think that juvenile diabetes may be caused by viruses, germs so tiny that you would need a special kind of microscope to see them. Colds and flu, measles and mumps are all virus diseases. People can easily catch these diseases from other people who have them. But diabetes doesn't work quite that way. You won't catch diabetes if you play with people who have it—not even if they sneeze on you.

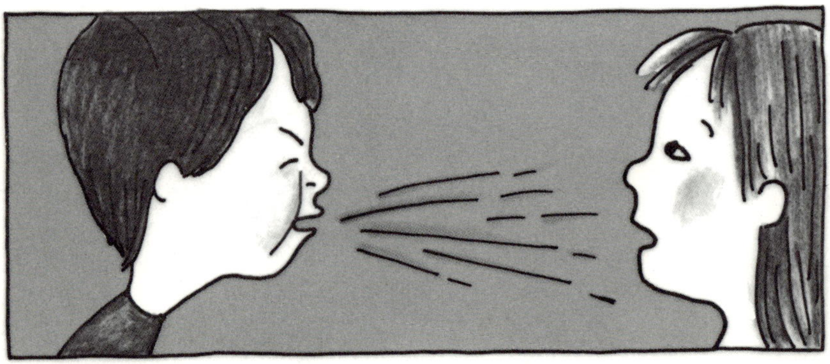

Apparently some of the same viruses that cause measles, mumps, and other diseases can also cause diabetes. The viruses may attack the pancreas and damage the cells that make insulin. Then they can't make their hormone. So when you eat, there is no insulin to make the sugars from foods go from the blood into the body cells. The sugar just stays in the blood.

There is another way a virus disease could hurt the pancreas. It happens by a sort of accident. When the body is attacked by a virus, it makes chemical defenses called antibodies. There are many different kinds of antibodies. There is one kind to match each virus. But sometimes a mistake happens. An antibody that matches a virus matches a body cell, too. Then antibodies of that kind don't just attack viruses. They can also hurt body cells.

When some people get a disease like mumps or measles, their bodies may make antibodies that attack cells in the pancreas. The antibodies would act as though these cells were dangerous germs. They would damage or kill the cells. Then the pancreas couldn't make enough insulin.

Most children get mumps or measles or other virus diseases. Yet most children ***don't*** get diabetes. Maybe they are just lucky enough not to make the wrong kind of antibodies. Or maybe it is a question of heredity. Children tend to be like their

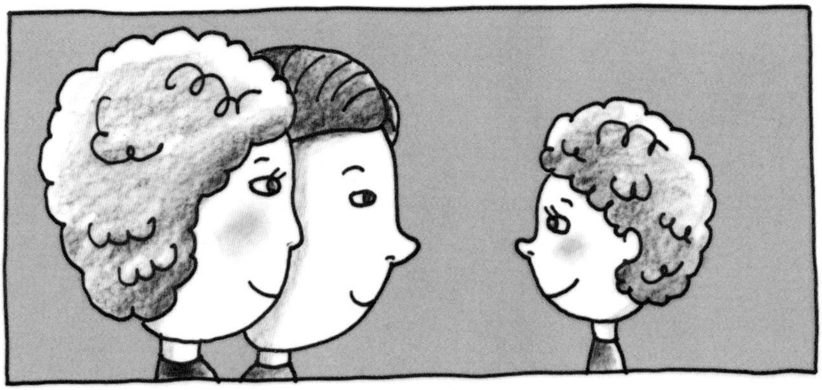

parents. You can inherit blue eyes or curly hair or a turned-up nose from your parents. Scientists think you can inherit an ability to get certain diseases, too. Diabetes is one of these diseases.

Children with juvenile diabetes can't make enough insulin. Some of them can't make any insulin at all.

Many grown-ups with diabetes have a different problem. They can make insulin. In fact, they have plenty of insulin in their blood. And yet, they still have too much sugar in their blood. What is wrong? Why doesn't their insulin work the way it should?

Scientists are trying to find out. They think one problem may be with the body cells. Insulin makes cells take in sugar. To do this, insulin has to hook onto the cells, on special little "hooks" called receptors. If the cells don't have enough of the right kind of receptors, insulin can't work on them. Scientists have found that many diabetics don't have enough receptors for insulin.

Another problem with diabetics may be too much glucagon, the hormone that makes the blood sugar go up. Their insulin can't keep the blood sugar level down because there is too much glucagon working against it.

How do you know if you have diabetes? Here are some danger signs:

You are thirsty all the time.

You have to make urine many times during the day and even at night, too.

You often feel weak and tired.

You feel hungry all the time.

You are losing weight, even though you eat a lot.

You get sores on your skin, and they take a long time to heal.

Things look fuzzy or double.

You have pains in your legs.

Anybody can have some of these warning signs without having diabetes. Maybe you are very thirsty because it is hot. Maybe you make a lot of urine because you drank some extra milk or soda. Your legs may ache after you do a lot of running

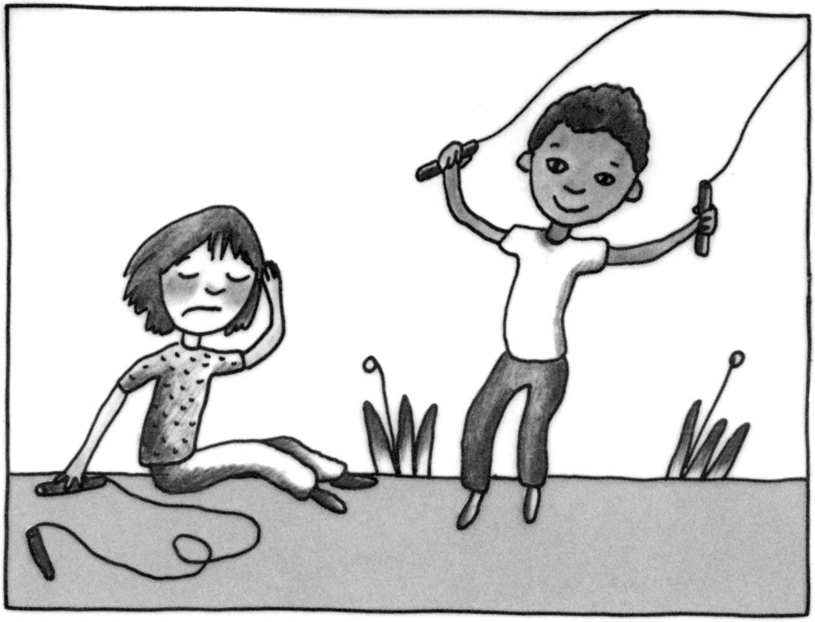

and jumping. Perhaps you feel tired because you haven't been getting enough sleep. But if you have many of these signs, and have them all the time, you should see a doctor.

Juvenile diabetes can appear very suddenly. A child may feel fine. Then, just a few weeks later, that same child may be so sick that he or she must be rushed to the hospital. Often juvenile diabetes first appears after an illness, like a cold or German measles.

In older people, diabetes may take years to develop. The person may hardly feel sick at all. In fact, people often find out they have diabetes when they are having their yearly checkup. The doctor finds sugar in their blood or urine.

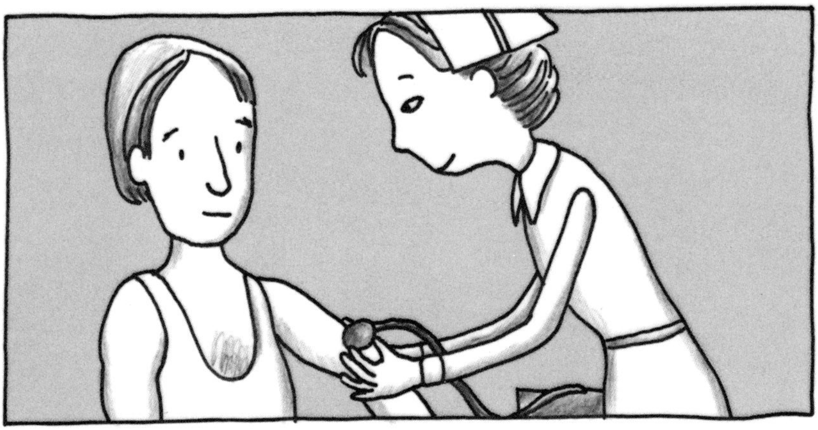

How does the sugar get into the urine? Urine is made in the kidneys. Each person has two kidneys, which are shaped like big kidney beans. Urine is one of the body's ways of getting rid of wastes.

It seems that whenever we do anything, we get waste products. Your family has its own waste products—old cans and bottles, scrap paper, apple cores and orange peels, dirty dishwater . . . You wash or flush some of these wastes down the drain. Others are put out for the garbage man to take away.

The body's waste products are chemicals. Blood carries these chemicals away from the body cells. All your blood flows through your kidneys, many times each day. The kidneys take out waste products from the blood. They also take out some water, to flush the wastes away. The mixture of water and wastes is urine. If there is too much of something in the blood, the kidneys take that out, too. Diabetics have too much sugar in their blood. So soon they have sugar in their urine, too.

When sugar passes into the urine, the urine gets thicker. Then more water goes from the blood into the urine. This water washes out other things, too.

Vitamins and minerals, proteins and fats are lost along with the sugar and water. What a mess!

Now we can see why those warning signs can be signs of diabetes. If you have diabetes, you have to make a lot of urine because your kidneys are getting rid of the extra sugar from the blood. You are thirsty all the time because you are losing so much water. You feel unusually weak and tired because your body can't use sugar for the energy it needs. You are hungry because you are losing so many good food materials, which are getting washed out in your urine.

If the sugar is not kept under control, other bad effects may develop. A diabetic is more likely than most people to get heart disease. High sugar levels may cause changes in the eyes. The person may go blind. High sugar levels may also causes changes in the nerves, which produce pain and numbness. Diabetics get infections easily, and they do not heal as quickly.

Urine tests for sugar are quick and easy. You could do it yourself. All you have to do is dip a special, chemically treated plastic strip into some of your urine and match the color of a spot to a chart to see if there is any sugar, and how much. (Other simple tests use tablets or tapes.) Some people find

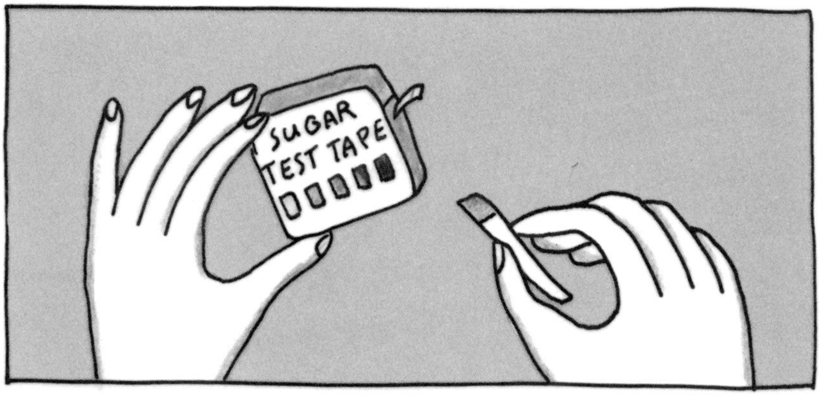

out they have diabetes when a urine test shows sugar. People with diabetes also test their urine every day, to see how well they are keeping it under control.

Blood tests for sugar are taken in a doctor's office or hospital. You may be a little scared the first time a nurse takes your blood for a test. But you soon get used to it. The blood is taken through a needle in your arm. It doesn't really hurt, and only a small amount of blood is needed for the tests. In fact, blood tests may also be done at home. Even a child can do them, getting enough blood for the tests by sticking a finger.

Sometimes the doctor tests the sugar in the blood early in the morning, before you have eaten anything. You may be given a thick sugar solution to drink. Then blood tests are taken every hour. That kind of test is used only when the doctor is not sure yet if the person has diabetes. It shows whether the pancreas is making enough insulin to put the sugar away in storage in the body cells.

What can you do about diabetes if you have it? It depends on what kind you have.

Many older people who get diabetes are fat. They eat too much, and they weigh too much. Their pancreas makes some insulin, but it is not enough to keep the body healthy. For these people, the best way to treat diabetes is to go on a diet. After they lose some weight, their pancreas will be making just the right amount of insulin.

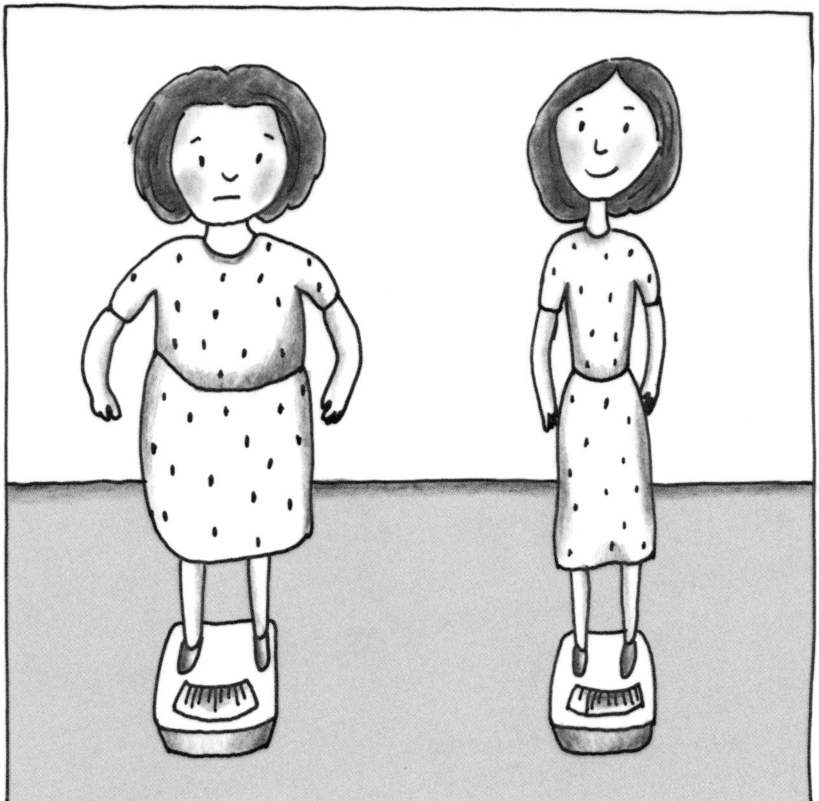

What is the right kind of diet for a diabetic? People used to think you had to cut out all sugars and starches. But that isn't necessary. It is a good idea, though, to cut out candy and drinks sweetened with sugar, as well as the fruits that are especially sugary. Get your sugars and starches mainly from

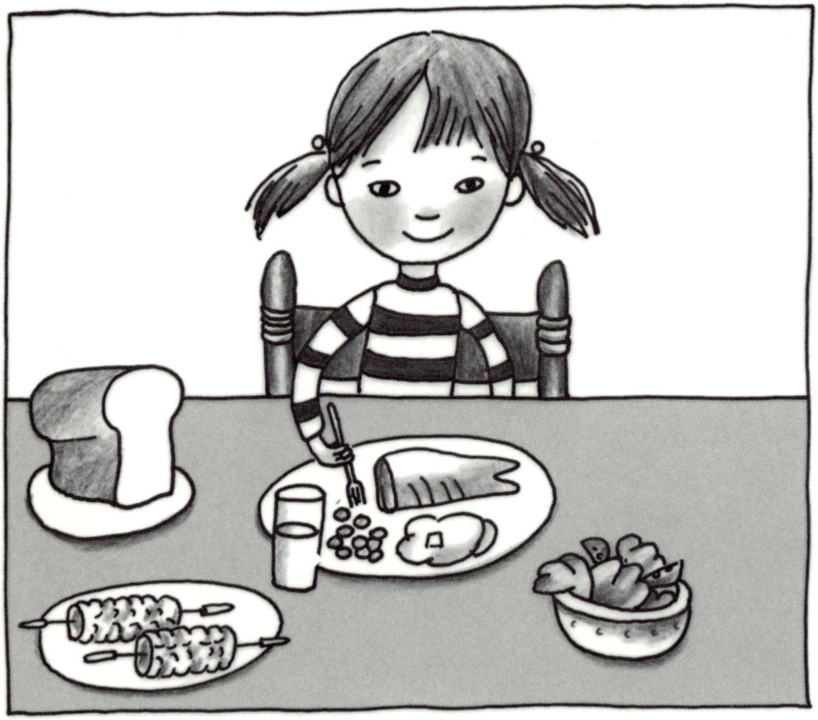

vegetables and whole-grain cereals and breads. Meat, fish, and other foods rich in protein are good, too. But a diabetic shouldn't eat too much animal fats. They may lead to heart disease, and that is something that many diabetics have trouble with anyway. The food should be enough to keep you healthy, but not enough to make you gain weight. This is a good kind of diet for both children and adults with diabetes. In fact, a good diet for a diabetic would be a healthy diet for anybody.

Some diabetics don't make enough insulin, even if they are the right weight. Nearly all juvenile diabetics don't make enough insulin of their own. They can take injections of insulin.

Does getting a shot at the doctor's upset you? Imagine getting injections every day, or even several times a day. Imagine giving injections to yourself! Once you get used to it, injections don't really hurt much. And giving yourself an injection is not too hard to do, once a doctor or nurse has taught

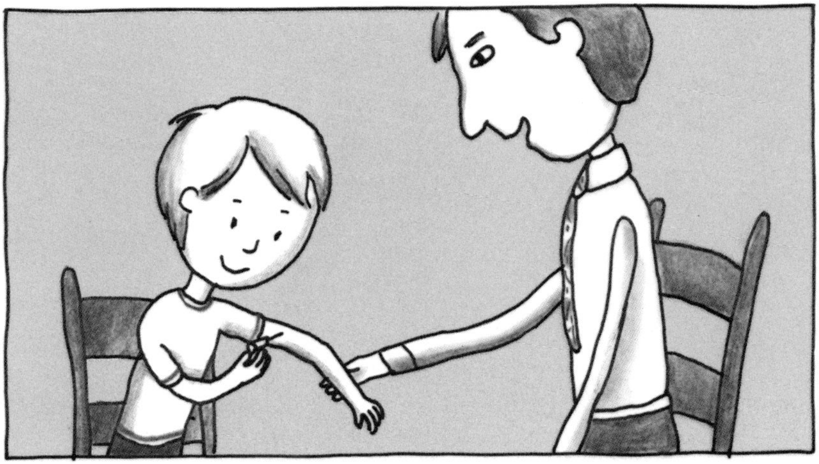

you how to do it properly. Children as young as four years old have been taught to give themselves insulin shots.

When you have diabetes, you have to be a sort of doctor's helper. You can call the doctor if there are any problems. But the doctor can't live with you. You and your family have to take charge of your daily treatment—taking sugar tests and giving insulin shots. Even if you are very young, you can learn to do both these things for yourself.

The insulin diabetics use comes from cattle and

pigs. There are several kinds. Some kinds of insulin start working right after you inject them, but they only work for a few hours. Then you need another shot. Other kinds of insulin take a long time to start working, but then they keep on working for twenty-four hours. A mixture of short- and long-acting insulin may be just right to keep the blood sugar level even. Each time you eat a meal, sugar goes into the blood. There must be insulin to bring the blood sugar level back down again.

If there is not enough insulin, the blood sugar goes up and up. The body starts to burn fats for energy. Ketone bodies are formed and start to poison the body. After a day or two, the person may fall unconscious. This condition is called a diabetic coma. If the person does not receive an injection of quick-acting insulin soon, he or she may die! That is why it is important for a diabetic to take sugar tests every day and call the doctor right away if the blood sugar is going up.

Too much insulin can also be dangerous. If the insulin shot is too strong, too much sugar will go out of the blood into the liver cells. Not enough sugar will go to the brain. Brain cells need a lot of energy. If they don't get enough sugar, they won't be able to work properly.

The reaction to too low a blood sugar level, caused by too much insulin, is called insulin shock. It can develop very quickly.

Sometimes diabetics take too much insulin by mistake. But sometimes even the right amount can cause a reaction. This might happen if you skip a meal. When you don't eat at the usual time, your blood sugar goes down. But if you are a diabetic taking insulin, you may already have taken your insulin shot for the day. You injected enough insulin to bring the blood sugar down to normal after a meal. But if you don't eat, there will be no extra sugar in your blood. Instead, insulin will take away some of the blood sugar your brain needs. So skipping a meal can cause an insulin reaction.

Taking snacks between meals and before exercising can help to avoid an insulin reaction. But for extra insurance, diabetics carry some hard candy or sugar cubes with them. If they feel dizzy and sick and think they might be getting an insulin reaction, they eat some sugar or candy, or drink a sweet drink. The extra sugar goes right into the blood and brings the level back to normal.

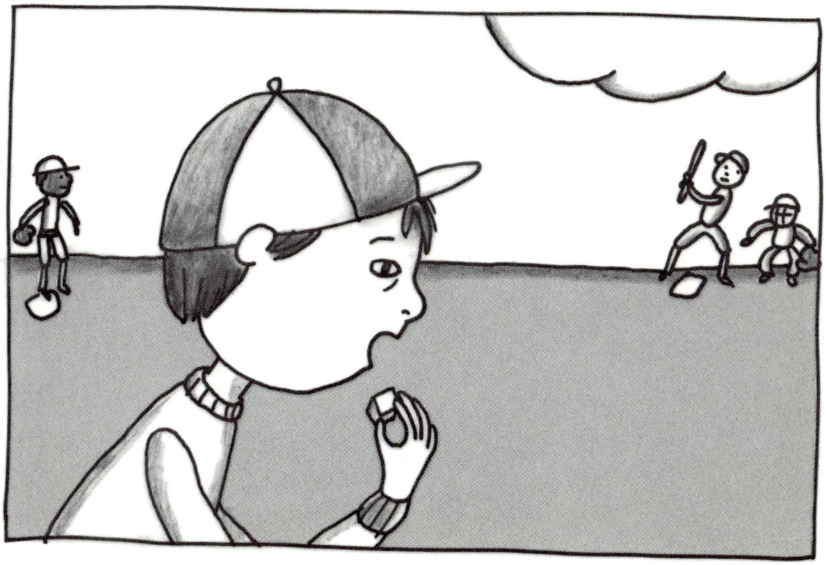

Here is how to tell the difference between a diabetic coma and an insulin reaction:

Insulin Reaction	*Diabetic Coma*
Starts suddenly	Develops gradually
Skin is pale and moist	Skin is dry and hot
Dizziness	No dizziness
Great hunger	Little hunger
Normal thirst	Great thirst
Shallow breathing	Deep, difficult breathing
Normal breath	Fruity smell on the breath
Tongue is moist	Tongue is dry
Normal urination	A lot of urine, with sugar
Confusion, acting strange	Sleepiness, tiredness

If you're still not sure what kind of reaction is developing, take some sugar. If that doesn't work in a few minutes, call the doctor right away.

Some people who have diabetes feel shy about telling others that they are diabetic. They may be ashamed to admit they are "different." But this is foolish. Everybody is different in various ways. When friends and relatives know someone has diabetes, they can be very helpful.

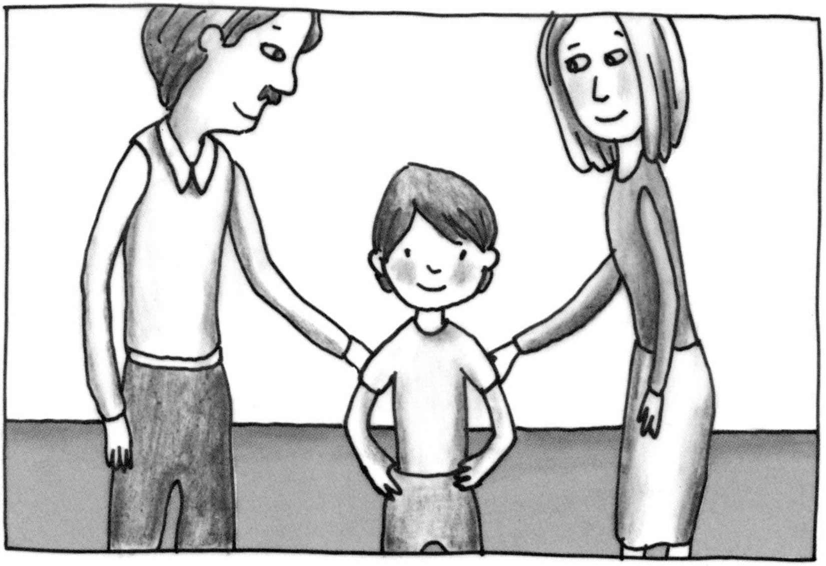

If you have a diabetic friend or parent, for example, you might help in spotting an insulin reaction early, before it becomes dangerous. If your diabetic friend suddenly seems confused, or starts laughing or crying for no reason, or acts strangely, you might suggest a candy bar. Sometimes friends notice the first signs of an insulin reaction before the diabetic realizes anything is wrong.

It is a good idea for diabetics to wear a special ID tag, so that people will know what to do to help if there is an emergency.

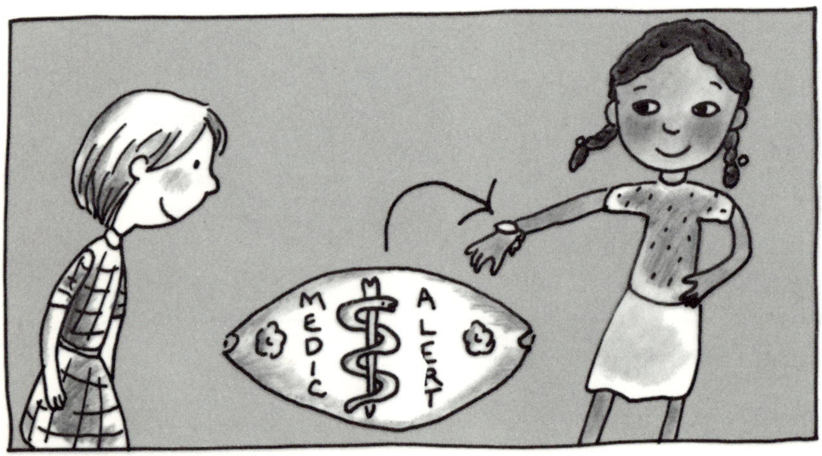

There are drugs that can help to control diabetes. These drugs do not need to be injected, like insulin. You can take them by swallowing a pill. Some of them work by making the pancreas produce more insulin. But they don't work on juvenile diabetics whose pancreas doesn't make any insulin at all, and they are not used for children.

Scientists are trying to find better ways to treat diabetes. They are trying to make better drugs, which will keep the blood sugar under better control and will not cause any harm to the body.

Some scientists are studying a hormone called somatostatin. This hormone does various things in the body. It works on the pancreas in two important ways. Somatostatin makes the pancreas produce less insulin. That doesn't sound very helpful for a diabetic. But somatostatin also makes the pancreas produce less glucagon, the hormone that makes blood sugar go up. An injection of somatostatin helps to bring diabetics' blood sugar level down.

Scientists are trying to make better forms of somatostatin, which will be more effective for diabetics.

Other researchers have developed ways to make human insulin. They think that would work better than insulin from cattle or pigs.

Other scientists are trying to build an artificial pancreas. They want to make a machine that can tell how much sugar is in the blood and send out just enough insulin to bring it down. That would be much better than giving an injection of insulin and then having to make sure to eat enough food and get just the right amount of exercise. With an artificial pancreas, a person wouldn't have to worry about getting an insulin reaction.

An artificial pancreas that works has already been built. The first models were as big as TV sets, too big to carry around. They are good for treating patients in the hospital. Newer models are about the size of a transistor radio, small enough to wear clipped to your belt. But these are only pumps that

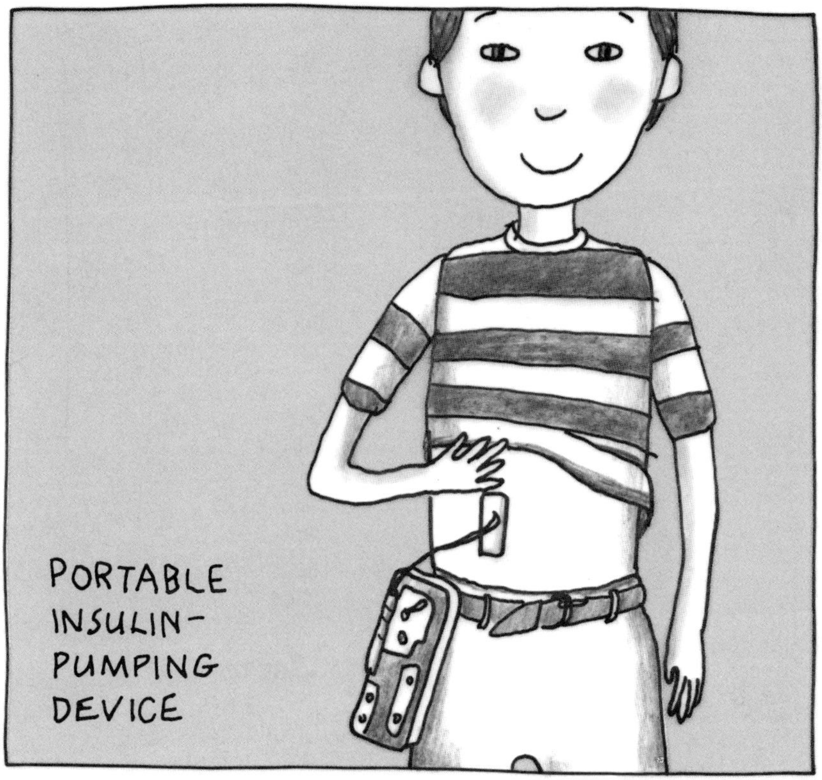

inject insulin into the blood. They do not measure the amount of sugar in the blood. Now scientists are trying to build a tiny artificial pancreas the size of a walnut, small enough to place inside a person's body.

Researchers are also trying to work out ways to transplant pancreas cells, so the body will be able to make its own insulin again.

All these studies may help diabetics in the future. But even today, by understanding their disease and taking measures to control it, diabetics can lead full and happy lives.

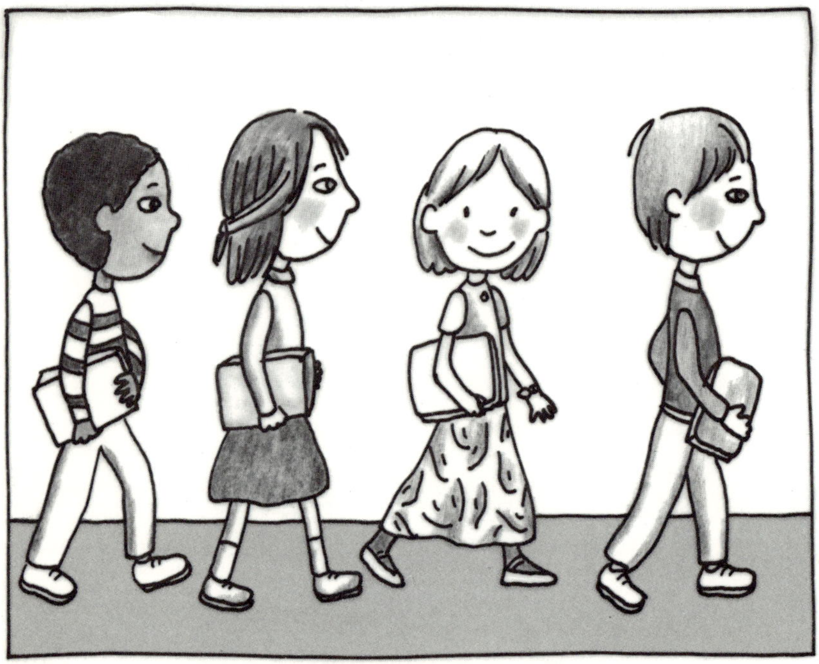

Here are some words you may want to use in talking about diabetes:

---

alpha cells: cells in the pancreas that produce glucagon.

beta cells: cells in the pancreas that produce insulin.

diabetes: a disease in which the body cannot use sugar properly.

diabetic coma: unconsciousness resulting from a large, uncontrolled rise in the amount of sugar in the blood. This can be dangerous.

fat: a high-energy food substance found in butter, oils, and meat.

glucagon: a hormone that increases the amount of sugar in the blood.

glucose: the most common kind of sugar in the blood. The body uses glucose for energy.

hormone: a body chemical that helps to control the work of the organs and systems. Insulin and glucagon are hormones that control the body's production and use of energy.

insulin: a hormone that decreases the amount of sugar in the blood and increases the storage of sugar in the liver.

insulin shock: a reaction to too much insulin in the blood. Dizziness, confusion, and unconsciousness may develop as the blood sugar level falls.

ketone bodies: chemicals that are formed when the body burns fats for energy.

pancreas: a gland that produces the hormones insulin and glucagon, as well as substances that help in the digestion of food.

protein: a food substance used mainly for building up body structures and keeping them healthy. It is found in foods like meat and eggs.

starch: a food substance found in bread, potatoes, and pasta that the body breaks down into sugars.

sugar: a quick-energy food substance found in fruits, candy, and soft drinks.

Silverstein, Alvin

Runaway sugar

L-Copy 1

DATE			
~~FEB 5 '90~~			
JAN 4 '94			